Made in United States
Troutdale, OR
10/11/2023

13612727R00086